NASM Essentials of
Personal Fitness Training

NASM™
NATIONAL ACADEMY OF SPORTS MEDICINE

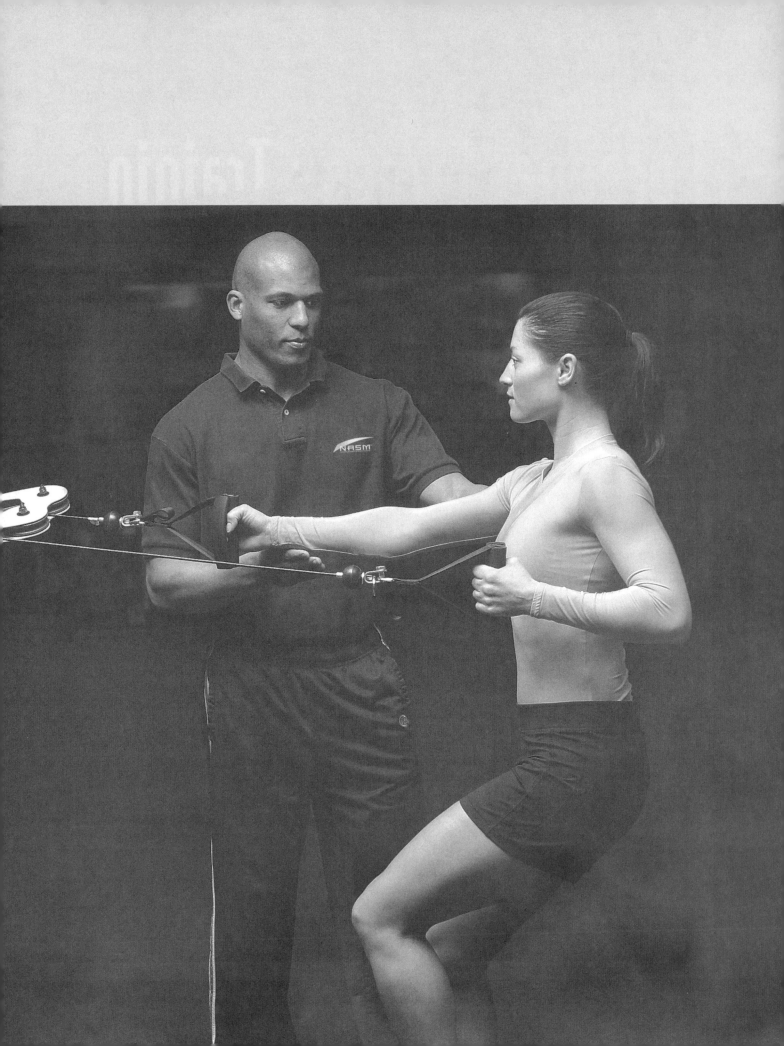

NASM Essentials of
Personal Fitness Training

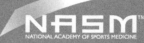

THIRD EDITION

Micheal A. Clark, DPT, MS, PES, CES
President and CEO
National Academy of Sports Medicine
Calabasas, CA

Scott C. Lucett, MS, PES, CES, CPT
Director of Education
National Academy of Sports Medicine
Calabasas, CA

Rodney J. Corn, MA, PES, CES, CPT
Training and Development Manager
National Academy of Sports Medicine
Calabasas, CA

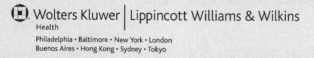
Wolters Kluwer | Lippincott Williams & Wilkins
Health
Philadelphia · Baltimore · New York · London
Buenos Aires · Hong Kong · Sydney · Tokyo

Acquisitions Editor: Emily Lupash
Managing Editor: Matthew J. Hauber
Marketing Manager: Christen D. Murphy
Production Editor: Jennifer P. Ajello
Designer: Risa Clow
Compositor: Techbooks
Printer: Victor Graphics

351 West Camden Street
Baltimore, MD 21201

530 Walnut Street
Philadelphia, PA 19106

Printed in the United States of America

Library of Congress Cataloging-in-Publication Data

Lucett, Scott.
    NASM essentials of personal fitness training : study guide / Scott Lucett. — 3rd ed.
        p. cm.
    ISBN 978-0-7817-7846-6 (alk. paper)
    1. Physical fitness—Vocational guidance—United States—Handbooks, manuals,
etc. 2. Health—Vocational guidance—United States—Handbooks, manuals, etc.
    I. National Academy of Sports Medicine. II. Title.
    GV481.L753 2008
    613.7—dc22

                                                            2007004408

To purchase additional copies of this book, call our customer service department at **(800) 638-3030**
or fax orders to **(301) 223-2320.** International customers should call **(301) 223-2300.**

Visit Lippincott Williams & Wilkins on the Internet: *http://www.LWW.com.* Lippincott Williams &
Wilkins customer service representatives are available from 8:30 am to 6:00 pm, EST.

07 08 09 10 11
1 2 3 4 5 6 7 8 9 10

Preface

INTRODUCTION TO THE COURSE

Welcome to the National Academy of Sports Medicine's Essentials of Personal Fitness Training home-study course. At NASM, our mission is to revolutionize the health and fitness industry by providing education, solutions, and tools that produce remarkable results. We aim to give health and fitness professionals an integrated approach to health, allowing them to guide others toward healthier lifestyles. Our educational continuum employs an easy-to-use, systematic approach in order to apply scientific and clinically accepted concepts.

HOW TO USE THIS STUDY GUIDE

This Study Guide is designed to help you master the basic concepts presented in the course. This study guide provides students with a way to evaluate their knowledge, strengths, and weaknesses through an interactive review process.

Simply follow the student daily planner in this study guide. For each study day, read the corresponding sections and complete the assignments listed. By following the student day planner, you will stay focused on key areas and studying will be simple. The planner has been carefully organized to break down scientific concepts into manageable sections. You may move at a faster pace if you desire, but we suggest following the planner to ensure proper mastery of all concepts.

STUDY TIPS

The most important characteristic for students to possess is a deep and passionate desire to learn.

That said, the following tips should help maximize the time spent on the course materials:

1. Pace yourself. You will be spending time watching presentations and demonstrations as well as reading the course text. Allow yourself enough time to get through the materials and thoroughly comprehend the information before progressing within the course.

2. Schedule your study time. Use the day planner provided in this workbook and fill in your specific study dates. Make sure to stick to them. This will ensure a reasonable timeframe for completing your work and certification examination.

3. Read and re-read. When reviewing the course text, scan the information once to obtain an overview of the material. Then, go back and read the information thoroughly.

4. Think about it. Stop frequently as you review course material to consider the concepts presented. Ask yourself how and when you can apply the techniques and information covered.

5. Lighten up. Use a highlighter to accent important concepts and information or areas that may require additional review and practice.

6. Do the exercises. Reading alone will probably not provide you with enough mastery of the material to pass the final examination. NASM strongly recommends going through each of the exercises in the study guide for each section after you have completed your reading.

7. Practice, practice, practice. Remember that the regular review and application of these principles is essential to your success. Apply what you've learned at every opportunity to help improve your techniques. Use the information you've uncovered to discuss and apply your knowledge to friends, clients, and relatives.

GETTING HELP

At NASM, your success is our success. We want to help in every way we can. The NASM staff is available to offer any assistance you may need throughout the course of your program. Whether you have technical or educational questions, we are available by phone and e-mail 8:00 A.M. to 5:00 P.M. (PST), Monday through Friday. Please call our toll-free number at 800.460.NASM or e-mail us questions at www.nasm.org.

SUCCESS PLAN

You have 120 days from your registration (date of purchase) to fully complete the course and take the final examination. Be sure to schedule your time accordingly! Use the following day planner to stay focused and track your progress. The day planner follows a 45-day reading and study plan. You do not need to work straight through for 45 days, but it is recommended that you do not take much time off between study sessions so that you will retain the material.

There are 45 full days of study material to get through. Average amounts of study time each day fall between one-half to a full hour. Make sure you have about 45 minutes to study on any given day. Sticking to the day planner will also give you ample time to prepare for the final exam before the 120-day expiration.

Study Day	Completion Date	Course Materials	Assignment
Day 1	_____ Fill in today's date	Front Matter and Chapter 1	▪ Read the Letter from the President ▪ Read the Code of Ethics ▪ Read Introduction ▪ Begin Reading Chapter 1
Day 2	_____ Date	Chapter 1	▪ Finish Reading Chapter 1 ▪ Watch Chapter 1 Presentation ▪ Perform Chapter 1 Exercises in the study guide
Day 3	_____ Date	Chapter 2	▪ Read Chapter 2
Day 4	_____ Date	Chapter 2	▪ Watch Chapter 2 Presentation ▪ Perform Chapter 2 Exercises in the study guide
Day 5	_____ Date	Chapter 3	▪ Read Chapter 3
Day 6	_____ Date	Chapter 3	▪ Watch Chapter 3 Presentation ▪ Perform Chapter 3 Exercises in the study guide
Day 7	_____ Date	Chapter 4	▪ Begin Reading Chapter 4
Day 8	_____ Date	Chapter 4	▪ Continue Reading Chapter 4
Day 9	_____ Date	Chapter 4	▪ Finish Reading Chapter 4
Day 10	_____ Date	Chapter 4	▪ Watch Chapter 4 Presentation ▪ Perform Chapter 4 Exercises in the study guide
Day 11	_____ Date	Chapter 5	▪ Begin Reading Chapter 5

Study Day	Completion Date	Course Materials	Assignment
Day 12	_____ *Date*	Chapter 5	▪ Continue Reading Chapter 5
Day 13	_____ *Date*	Chapter 5	▪ Finish Reading Chapter 5
Day 14	_____ *Date*	Chapter 5	▪ Watch Chapter 5 Presentation ▪ Perform Chapter 5 Exercises in the study guide
Day 15	_____ *Date*	Chapter 6	▪ Begin Reading Chapter 6
Day 16	_____ *Date*	Chapter 6	▪ Continue Reading Chapter 6
Day 17	_____ *Date*	Chapter 6	▪ Finish Reading Chapter 6
Day 18	_____ *Date*	Chapter 6	▪ Watch Chapter 6 Presentation ▪ Perform Chapter 6 Exercises in the study guide
Day 19	_____ *Date*	Chapter 7	▪ Begin Reading Chapter 7
Day 20	_____ *Date*	Chapter 7	▪ Finish Reading Chapter 7
Day 21	_____ *Date*	Chapter 7	▪ Watch Chapter 7 Presentation ▪ Perform Chapter 7 Exercises in the study guide
Day 22	_____ *Date*	Chapter 8	▪ Read Chapter 8
Day 23	_____ *Date*	Chapter 8	▪ Watch Chapter 8 Presentation ▪ Perform Chapter 8 Exercises in the study guide
Day 24	_____ *Date*	Chapter 9	▪ Read Chapter 9
Day 25	_____ *Date*	Chapter 9	▪ Watch Chapter 9 Presentation ▪ Perform Chapter 9 Exercises in the study guide
Day 26	_____ *Date*	Chapter 10	▪ Read Chapter 10 ▪ Watch Chapter 10 Presentation ▪ Perform Chapter 10 Exercises in the study guide
Day 27	_____ *Date*	Chapter 11	▪ Read Chapter 11 ▪ Watch Chapter 11 Presentation ▪ Perform Chapter 11 Exercises in the study guide
Day 27	_____ *Date*	Chapter 12	▪ Read Chapter 12
Day 28	_____ *Date*	Chapter 12	▪ Watch Chapter 12 Presentation ▪ Perform Chapter 12 Exercises in the study guide
Day 29	_____ *Date*	Chapter 13	▪ Begin Reading Chapter 13
Day 30	_____ *Date*	Chapter 13	▪ Finish Reading Chapter 13
Day 31	_____ *Date*	Chapter 13	▪ Watch Chapter 13 Presentation ▪ Perform Chapter 13 Exercises in the study guide

Study Day	Completion Date	Course Materials	Assignment
Day 32	_____ *Date*	Chapter 14	▪ Begin Reading Chapter 14
Day 33	_____ *Date*	Chapter 14	▪ Continue Reading Chapter 14
Day 34	_____ *Date*	Chapter 14	▪ Finish Reading Chapter 14
Day 35	_____ *Date*	Chapter 14	▪ Watch Chapter 14 Presentation ▪ Perform Chapter 14 Exercises in the study guide
Day 36	_____ *Date*	Chapter 15	▪ Begin Reading Chapter 15
Day 37	_____ *Date*	Chapter 15	▪ Finish Reading Chapter 15
Day 38	_____ *Date*	Chapter 15	▪ Watch Chapter 15 Presentation ▪ Perform Chapter 15 Exercises in the study guide
Day 39	_____ *Date*	Chapter 16	▪ Read Chapter 16 ▪ Watch Chapter 16 Presentation ▪ Perform Chapter 16 Exercises in the study guide
Day 40	_____ *Date*	Chapter 17	▪ Read Chapter 17
Day 41	_____ *Date*	Chapter 17	▪ Watch Chapter 17 Presentation ▪ Perform Chapter 17 Exercises in the study guide
Day 42	_____ *Date*	Chapter 18	▪ Read Chapter 18
Day 43	_____ *Date*	Chapter 18	▪ Watch Chapter 18 Presentation ▪ Perform Chapter 18 Exercises in the study guide
Day 44	_____ *Date*	Review	▪ Review all of your chapter exercises ▪ Make note of any questions you got wrong ▪ Review those sections in the text
Day 45	_____ *Date*	Practice Exam	▪ Take the online Practice Exam (www.nasm.org) ▪ After you have finished, review any sections that you had trouble with
Finish	_____ *Date*	Final Exam	▪ Take the Final Exam and become an NASM Certified Personal Trainer!

Take out a monthly calendar now and fill in the exact dates that correspond to your study schedule. Filling in your exact study dates is a good way to plan ahead for days that you know you will be unable to study, so that you do not fall behind. If, at any point, you feel you've lost momentum, use the above study tips to get back on track.

Contents

The Scientific Rationale for Integrated Training

STUDY GUIDE EXERCISES

Exercise 1-1: Essential Vocabulary

First, skim through Chapter 1 of the text. Then, fully read through Chapter 1 and watch the presentations for Chapter 1. As you read and review, find and highlight the vocabulary words numbered below.

The purpose of this exercise is to have an understanding of key terms utilized in the section. Without referring back to the text, match the terms with their proper definitions.

VOCABULARY WORDS

1. _____ Deconditioned

2. _____ Proprioception

3. _____ Proprioceptively enriched environment

4. _____ Phase of training

5. _____ Stabilization

6. _____ Neuromuscular efficiency

7. _____ Prime mover

8. _____ Rate of force production

9. _____ Superset

DEFINITION

A. An unstable (but controlled) environment where exercises are performed that causes the body to use its internal balance and stabilization mechanisms.

B. How quickly a muscle can generate force.

C. Ability of the body's stabilizing muscles to provide support for joints as well as maintain posture and balance during movement.

D. Smaller divisions of training progressions that fall within the three building blocks of training.

E. A state of lost physical fitness, which may include muscle imbalances, decreased flexibility, and/or a lack of core and joint stability.

F. Set of two exercises that are performed back-to-back without any rest time between them.

G. The muscle that acts as the main source of motive movement.

H. The cumulative neural input to the central nervous system from mechanoreceptors that sense position and limb movement.

I. The ability of the body's nerves to effectively send messages to the body's muscles.

Exercise 1-2: Short Answer

Review the information in Chapter 1. Now, answer the following question in one or two sentences.

OVERVIEW OF THE PERSONAL TRAINING INDUSTRY

Briefly describe past, present, and future training trends and how this evolution directly affects health and fitness professionals today.

_____

_____

_____

_____

_____

Exercise 1-3: Understanding Training Goals

After your review of the Strength Training section in Chapter 1, write out the goals of each phase listed below. Your answers do not have to be technical. In fact, write like you would speak to a new prospect who is inquiring about training.

Phase 2: Strength Endurance

_____

_____

_____

Phase 3: Hypertrophy

_____

_____

_____

Phase 4: Maximal Strength

_____

_____

_____

After your review of the Power Training section in Chapter 1, write out the goals of the phase listed at the top of the next page. Your answers do not have to be technical.

   In fact, write like you would speak to a new prospect who is inquiring about training.

Phase 5: Power

_____

_____

_____

CHAPTER 1 — ANSWER KEY

Exercise 1-1 Answers

1. E   3. A   5. C   7. G   9. F
2. H   4. D   6. I   8. B

Exercise 1-2 Answers

The typical client of the past was probably better prepared for activity in the gym as a result of an environment that required more daily activity.

The client of the present is surrounded by a wealth of technology and automation. This has begun to take a toll on public health, leading to dysfunction and increased injury. The new mindset in fitness should cater to creating programs that address functional capacity as part of a safe program designed especially for each individual person.

Exercise 1-3 Answers

1. Phase 2: Strength Endurance
   Enhance stabilization strength and endurance while increasing prime mover strength.
2. Phase 3: Hypertrophy
   Designed for individuals who have the goal of maximal muscle hypertrophy.
3. Phase 4: Maximal Strength
   Works toward the goal of increasing maximal prime mover strength.
4. Phase 5: Power
   Enhances prime mover strength while also improving the rate of force production (how quickly a muscle can generate force).

Basic Exercise Science

STUDY GUIDE EXERCISES

Exercise 2-1: Essential Vocabulary

First, skim through Chapter 2 of the text. Then, fully read through Chapter 2 and watch the presentations for Chapter 2. As you read, find and highlight the vocabulary words numbered below.

The purpose of this exercise is to have an understanding of key terms utilized in the section. Without referring back to the text, match the terms with their proper definitions.

VOCABULARY WORDS

1. _____ Kinetic chain

2. _____ Nervous system

3. _____ Sensory function

4. _____ Integrative function

5. _____ Motor function

6. _____ Neuron

7. _____ Sensory (afferent) neurons

8. _____ Interneurons

9. _____ Motor (efferent) neurons

10. _____ Central nervous system

11. _____ Peripheral nervous system

12. _____ Mechanoreceptors

DEFINITION

A. Cranial and spinal nerves that spread throughout the body and serve to relay information from bodily organs to the brain and from the brain to bodily organs.

B. Neurons that transmit nerve impulses from effector sites to the brain or spinal cord.

C. Organs sensitive to change in tension of the muscle and the rate of that change.

D. The neuromuscular response to sensory information.

E. The combination and interrelation of the nervous, skeletal, and muscular systems.

F. The functional unit of the nervous system.

G. Large groups of cells that form nerves, which provide a communication network within the body.

H. The ability of the nervous system to sense changes in either internal or external environments.

I. Neurons that transmit impulses from one neuron to another.

J. Consists of the brain and spinal cord and serves mainly to interpret information.

K. The ability of the nervous system to analyze and interpret sensory information to allow for proper decision making, which produces the appropriate response.

13. _____ Muscle spindles

14. _____ Golgi tendon organs

15. _____ Joint receptors

L. Neurons that transmit nerve impulses from the brain or spinal cord to the effector sites.

M. Sensory receptors responsible for sensing distortion in bodily tissues.

N. Receptors sensitive to pressure, acceleration, and deceleration in the joint.

O. Fibers sensitive to change in length of the muscle and the rate of that change.

Exercise 2-2: Knowledge of Terms

After reading Chapter 2, use any of the following terms to fill in the blanks below:

Muscular system

Muscle

Tendons

Sarcomere

Neural activation

Neurotransmitter

Pennation

1. _____ attach muscles to bone and provide the anchor from which the muscle can exert force and control the bone and joint.

2. _____ is tissue consisting of long cells that contract when stimulated to produce motion.

3. _____ are chemical messengers that transmit electrical impulses from the nerve to the muscle.

4. The _____ is a series of muscles that the nervous system commands to move the skeletal system.

5. The functional unit of muscle that produces muscular contraction (which consists of repeating sections of actin and myosin) is called the _____.

6. The arrangement of muscle fibers that run at an angle to the tendon is called _____.

7. _____ is the contraction of a muscle generated by the communication between the nervous system and muscular system.

Exercise 2-3: Essential Vocabulary

Without referring back to the text, match the terms with their proper definitions.

VOCABULARY WORDS

1. _____ Skeletal system

2. _____ Bones

3. _____ Joints

4. _____ Axial skeleton

5. _____ Appendicular skeleton

6. _____ Depression

7. _____ Process

8. _____ Arthrokinematics

9. _____ Synovial joints

10. _____ Nonsynovial joints

11. _____ Ligament

DEFINITION

A. The movable places where two or more bones meet.

B. Portion of the skeletal system that includes the upper and lower extremities.

C. Projection protruding from the bone where muscles, tendons, and ligaments can attach.

D. The body's frame, which is comprised of bones and joints.

E. Portion of the skeletal system that consists of the skull, rib cage, and vertebral column.

F. The movements of the joints.

G. Connective tissue that connects bone to bone.

H. Joints that are held together by a joint capsule and ligaments and are most associated with movement in the body.

I. Hard connective tissues that connect to create a skeletal framework.

J. Flattened or indented portion of bone, which can be a muscle attachment site.

K. Joints that do not have a joint cavity, connective tissue, or cartilage.

Exercise 2-4: Characteristics of Muscle Fiber Types

Review the muscle-fiber information in Chapter 2. Note which of the following choices would be a characteristic of type I and which would be a characteristic of type II.

1. Lower in capillaries, mitochondria, and myoglobin _____

2. Smaller in size _____

3. Produce less force _____

4. Slow to fatigue _____

5. Long-term contractions _____

6. Produce more force _____

7. Quick to fatigue _____

8. Short-term contractions (force and power) _____

CHAPTER 2 — ANSWER KEY

Exercise 2-1 Answers

1. E	4. K	7. B	10. J	13. O
2. G	5. D	8. I	11. A	14. C
3. H	6. F	9. L	12. M	15. N

Exercise 2-2 Answers

1. Tendons
2. Muscle
3. Neurotransmitters
4. Muscular system
5. Sarcomere
6. Pennation
7. Neural activation

Exercise 2-3 Answers

1. D	4. E	7. C	10. K
2. I	5. B	8. F	11. G
3. A	6. J	9. H	

Exercise 2-4 Answers

1. Type II
2. Type I
3. Type I
4. Type I
5. Type I
6. Type II
7. Type II
8. Type II

3

The Cardiorespiratory System

STUDY GUIDE EXERCISES

Exercise 3-1: Essential Vocabulary

First, skim through Chapter 3 of the text. Then, fully read through Chapter 3 and watch the presentations for Chapter 3 of the text. As you read, find and highlight the vocabulary words numbered below.

The purpose of this exercise is to have an understanding of key terms utilized in the section. Without referring back to the text, match the terms with their proper definitions.

VOCABULARY WORDS

1. _____ Cardiorespiratory system

2. _____ Cardiovascular system

3. _____ Heart

4. _____ Blood

5. _____ Blood vessel

6. _____ Arteries

7. _____ Veins

8. _____ Capillaries

DEFINITION

A. Muscular pump that rhythmically contracts to push blood throughout the body.

B. Acts as a medium to deliver and collect essential products to and from the tissues of the body.

C. A system comprised of the cardiovascular and respiratory systems.

D. A hollow tube that allows blood to be transported to and from the heart.

E. The smallest blood vessel that is the location where substances such as oxygen, nutrients, hormones, and waste products are exchanged between tissues.

F. Vessels that transport blood back to the heart.

G. Comprised of the heart, the blood it pumps, and the blood vessels that transport the blood from the heart to the tissues of the body.

H. Vessels that transport blood away from the heart.

Exercise 3-2: Knowledge of Terms

After reading Chapter 3, use any of the following terms to fill in the blanks below:

Heart

70–80 beats per minute

75–80 mL per beat

Cardiovascular system

Mediastinum

Ventricles

Atriums

1. The _____ is comprised of four hollow chambers that are delineated into interdependent pumps on either side.

2. _____ are chambers located inferiorly on either side of the heart.

3. The heart rate of the typical person is approximately _____.

4. The _____ is comprised of the heart, the blood it pumps, and the blood vessels that transport the blood from the heart to the tissues of the body.

Exercise 3-3: Essential Vocabulary

Without referring back to the text, match the terms with their proper definitions.

VOCABULARY WORDS

1. _____ Respiratory system

2. _____ Inspiration

3. _____ Expiration

4. _____ Aerobic

5. _____ Anaerobic

6. _____ Bioenergetics

7. _____ Adenosine triphosphate

DEFINITION

A. The exhalation of air during the process of breathing.

B. Looks at how chemical energy is converted into mechanical energy.

C. An action that occurs in the presence of oxygen.

D. Cellular structure that serves as a storage and transfer unit within the cells of the body for energy.

E. A system including the lungs and their nervous and circulatory supply that collects oxygen from the external environment and transports it to the blood stream.

F. The inhalation of air during the process of breathing.

G. An action that is not dependent on oxygen for proper execution.

Exercise 3-4: Short Answer

Review the information in Chapter 3. Now, answer the following questions in one or two sentences.

1. How does the cardiorespiratory system relate to human movement?

_____

_____

2. How is oxygen related to energy expenditure?

_____

_____

3. How can dysfunctional breathing (chest breathing) have ill effects on the kinetic chain?

_____

_____

CHAPTER 3 — ANSWER KEY

Exercise 3-1 Answers

1. C	3. A	5. D	7. F
2. G	4. B	6. H	8. E

Exercise 3-2 Answers

1. Heart	3. 70–80 beats per minute
2. Ventricles	4. Cardiovascular system

Exercise 3-3 Answers

1. E	3. A	5. G	7. D
2. F	4. C	6. B	

Exercise 3-4 Answers

1. The cardiorespiratory system provides the kinetic chain with essential elements such as oxygen to help sustain activity or recover from it.
2. Oxygen is the necessary catalyst for aerobic activity that is prolonged for periods >30 seconds allowing for greater caloric expenditure.
3. Dysfunctional breathing associated with stress and/or anxiety becomes shallower and utilizes more secondary muscles more predominantly than the diaphragm. These secondary muscles all connect directly to the cervical and cranial portions of the body. Their increased activity leads to the restriction of the joints in that region, which leads to improper movement and further dysfunction.

Human Movement Science

STUDY GUIDE EXERCISES

Exercise 4-1: Essential Vocabulary

First, skim through Chapter 4 of the text. Then, fully read through Chapter 4 and watch the presentations for Chapter 4. As you read, find and highlight the vocabulary words numbered below.

The purpose of this exercise is to have an understanding of key terms utilized in the section. Without referring back to the text, match the terms with their proper definitions.

VOCABULARY WORDS

1. _____ Biomechanics
2. _____ Eccentric
3. _____ Isometric
4. _____ Concentric
5. _____ Length-tension relationship
6. _____ Force-couple
7. _____ Proprioception
8. _____ Sensorimotor integration
9. _____ Motor control
10. _____ Knowledge of performance

DEFINITION

A. Refers to the length at which a muscle can produce the greatest force.
B. Muscle action where there is no appreciable change in muscle length.
C. Information that the nervous system utilizes to gather information about the environment to produce movement.
D. Synergistic action of muscles to produce movement around a joint.
E. When a muscle exerts more force than is being placed on it, which leads to the shortening of the muscle.
F. Ability of nervous system to gather and interpret information and select and execute the proper motor response.
G. The study of how the kinetic chain creates movements.
H. When a muscle exerts less force than is being placed upon it, which results in the lengthening of a muscle.
I. Provides information about the quality of a movement during an exercise.
J. The study of how internal and external forces affect the way the body moves.

Exercise 4-2: Knowledge of Terms

After reading Chapter 4, write in the appropriate definitions, in your own words.

Sagittal plane

_____

_____

Frontal plane

_____

_____

Transverse plane

_____

_____

Refer back to Chapter 2 for a review of the following terms. Write in the appropriate definitions, in your own words.

Agonists

_____

_____

Synergists

_____

_____

Stabilizers

_____

_____

Antagonists

_____

_____

Exercise 4-3: Knowledge of Movement

Complete the following exercises to reinforce what you have just read. Choose the correct answer for each of the following questions by referring to the picture at the top of the next page (you may want to refer back to Chapter 2 to review the definition of agonists, antagonists, synergists, and stabilizers).

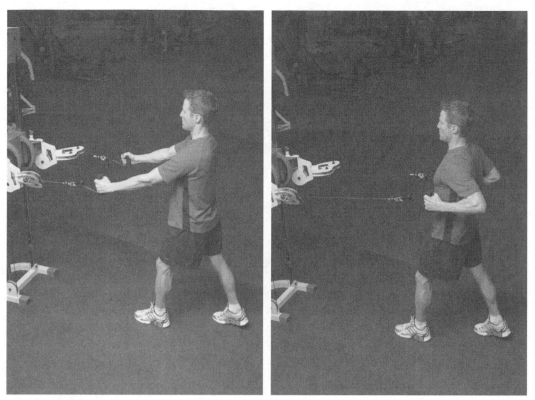

Standing Cable Row

1. In which plane of motion is this exercise occurring?
   Sagittal
   Frontal
   Transverse

2. What motion is occurring at the shoulder joint during the concentric phase?
   Abduction
   Adduction
   Extension

3. Which muscle is the agonist in this motion at the shoulder joint?
   Latissimus dorsi
   Triceps
   Rhomboids

4. Which muscle is the antagonist in this motion at the shoulder joint?
   Pectoralis major
   Posterior deltoid
   Biceps

5. Which muscle is a synergist in this motion at the shoulder joint?
   Anterior deltoid
   Pectoralis major
   Posterior deltoid

6. Which muscle(s) stabilize this motion at the shoulder joint?
   Rotator cuff
   Bicep
   Tricep

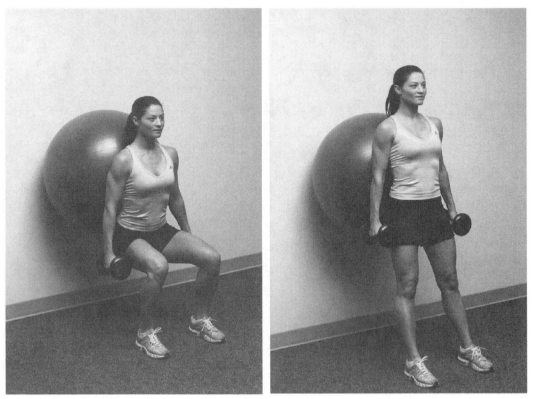

Ball Squat

7. Which plane of motion is this exercise occurring in?
   Sagittal
   Frontal
   Transverse

8. What motion is occurring at the hip during the concentric phase?
   Flexion
   Extension
   Adduction

9. Which muscle is the agonist in this motion at the hip?
   Hamstring
   Psoas
   Gluteus maximus

10. Which muscle is the antagonist in this motion at the hip?
    Psoas
    Quadriceps
    Hamstring

11. Which muscle is a synergist in this motion at the hip?
    Hamstring
    Psoas
    Gluteus maximus

12. Which muscle(s) stabilize this motion?
    Psoas
    Gluteus maximus
    Transversus abdominis

Exercise 4-4: Knowledge of Action

Complete the following exercise to reinforce what you have just read. Review the following table and write in the appropriate missing words. Check your answers before moving on to the next exercise.

Action	Performance
Eccentric	_____
	Decelerates and/or reduces force
Isometric	_____
	Dynamically stabilizes force
Concentric	Moving in the opposite direction of the resistance
	_____ and/or produces force

Exercise 4-5: Observation

Refer back to the anatomy portion of the chapter to complete the following exercise. Fill in the best answer for each of the following questions.

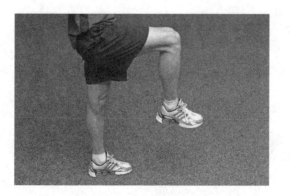

Name one or two primary muscle(s) that perform(s) the following actions:

1. Accelerate hip flexion:

_____

2. Decelerate hip flexion:

_____

3. Stabilize the hip:

_____

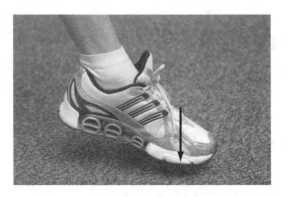

Name one or two primary muscle(s) that perform(s) the following actions:

4. Accelerate plantar flexion:

_____

5. Decelerate plantar flexion:

_____

6. Stabilize the foot and ankle:

_____

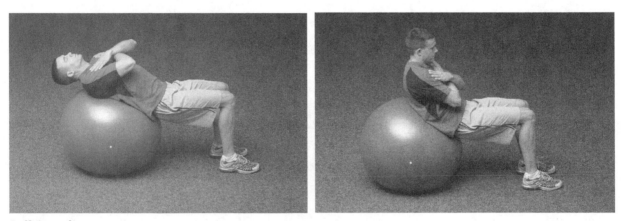

Ball Crunch

Name one or two primary muscle(s) that perform(s) the following actions:

7. Accelerate spinal flexion:

_____

8. Decelerate spinal extension:

_____

9. Stabilizes the spine:

_____

CHAPTER 4 — ANSWER KEY

Exercise 4-1 Answers

1. J   4. E   7. C   10. I
2. H   5. A   8. F
3. B   6. D   9. G

Exercise 4-2 Answers

Sagittal plane: Bisects the body to create right and left halves. Movements include flexion and extension.

Frontal plane: Bisects the body to create front and back halves. Movements include abduction and adduction of the limbs, lateral flexion of the spine, and eversion and inversion of the foot ankle complex.

Transverse plane: Bisects the body to create upper and lower halves. Movements include internal and external rotation for the limbs, right and left rotation for the head and trunk, and radioulnar pronation and supination.

Agonists: Muscles most responsible for a particular movement.

Synergists: Assists agonists during a movement.

Stabilizers: Muscles that support the body while other muscles are performing movement.

Antagonists: Muscles that oppose the agonist muscles.

Exercise 4-3 Answers

1. Sagittal
2. Extension
3. Latissimus dorsi
4. Pectoralis major
5. Posterior deltoid
6. Rotator cuff
7. Sagittal
8. Extension
9. Gluteus maximus
10. Psoas
11. Hamstring
12. Transversus abdominis

Exercise 4-4 Answers

Action	Performance
Eccentric	**Moving in the same direction as the resistance**
	Decelerates and/or reduces force
Isometric	**No visible movement with or against resistance**
	Dynamically stabilizes force
Concentric	Moving in the opposite direction of the resistance
	Accelerates and/or produces force

Exercise 4-5 Answers

1. Psoas, rectus femoris, tensor fascia latae
2. Gluteus maximus, hamstring
3. Transversus abdominis, adductors, gluteus medius
4. Gastrocnemius, soleus
5. Anterior tibialis
6. Peroneus Longus
7. Rectus abdominis, obliques
8. Rectus abdominis, obliques
9. Transversus abdominis

Fitness Assessment

STUDY GUIDE EXERCISES

Exercise 5-1: Essential Vocabulary

First, skim through Chapter 5 of the text. Then, fully read through Chapter 5 and watch the presentations for Chapter 5. As you read, find and highlight the vocabulary words numbered below.

The purpose of this exercise is to have an understanding of key terms utilized in the section. Without referring back to the text, match the terms with their proper definitions.

VOCABULARY WORDS

1. _____ Integrated fitness assessment

2. _____ Structural efficiency

3. _____ PAR-Q

4. _____ Objective information

5. _____ Postural equilibrium

6. _____ Diastolic pressure

7. _____ Posture

8. _____ Subjective information

9. _____ Functional efficiency

10. _____ Systolic pressure

DEFINITION

A. Ability of the neuromuscular system to monitor and manipulate movement using the least amount of energy, creating the least amount of stress on the kinetic chain.

B. Signifies the minimum pressure within the arteries through a full cardiac cycle.

C. The ability to efficiently maintain balance.

D. Feedback from the client to the fitness professional regarding personal history.

E. Provides the fitness professional with a three-dimensional representation of the client, which enables proper construction of a training program.

F. Measurable data that can be utilized to denote improvements in the client, as well as the effectiveness of the program.

G. Alignment and function of the kinetic chain at any given moment.

H. Alignment of the musculoskeletal system that allows a center of gravity to be maintained over a base of support.

I. Reflects the pressure produced by the heart as it pumps blood to the body.

J. Questionnaire that is designed to help qualify clients for activity levels and identify those who may need medical attention.

Exercise 5-2: Practical Application—Physiological Assessments

After reading Chapter 5, complete the following exercises to practice what you have just read.

CALCULATING HEART RATE ZONES

Complete the following section to determine your heart rate zones.

Step One—Maximum Heart Rate
In the space given, write your maximum heart rate and the formula you utilized to determine it.
Formula: _____
Maximum Heart Rate: _____

Step Two—Personal Training Zones
Complete the following chart to determine your training heart rate zones, utilizing the maximum heart rate you determined in Step One.

Maximum Heart Rate × 0.65 equals Maximum Heart Rate × 0.75 = _____

Maximum Heart Rate × 0.80 equals Maximum Heart Rate × 0.85 = _____

Maximum Heart Rate × 0.86 equals Maximum Heart Rate × 0.90 = _____

Step Three—Training Zones of Others
After completing your heart rate training ranges, practice utilizing this method on other fitness professionals and/or clients. (These same participants will be utilized for further assessments.)

Name: _____

Maximum Heart Rate: _____

Maximum Heart Rate × 0.65 equals Maximum Heart Rate × 0.75 = _____

Maximum Heart Rate × 0.80 equals Maximum Heart Rate × 0.85 = _____

Maximum Heart Rate × 0.86 equals Maximum Heart Rate × 0.90 = _____

Name: _____

Maximum Heart Rate: _____

Maximum Heart Rate × 0.65 equals Maximum Heart Rate × 0.75 = _____

Maximum Heart Rate × 0.80 equals Maximum Heart Rate × 0.85 = _____

Maximum Heart Rate × 0.86 equals Maximum Heart Rate × 0.90 = _____

Exercise 5-3: Practical Application—Cardiorespiratory Assessments

Read through Chapter 5 and complete the following exercises:

STEP TEST

Using yourself or one of the participants from Exercise 5-3, complete the
Step Test, following instructions given in the chapter. (Remember that Step One of the Step Test has already been completed.)

Complete the following information after completion of the Step Test. Refer to the text to locate the category and determine which zone would be an appropriate starting point for the participant.

Participant Name: _____

Recorded pulse for 30 seconds _____ = "recovery pulse"

Duration of the exercise (sec) × 100

Recovery pulse × 5.6 = _____

Category: _____

Starting zone:

Exercise 5-4: Observation

Read through Chapter 5 and complete the following exercises:

DYNAMIC POSTURAL ASSESSMENTS

With a client or fitness professional, perform the following movement observations, utilizing the given charts. Only check gross deviations. This exercise is to offer hands-on practice with observing movement and the kinetic chain checkpoints.

Overhead Squat

INSTRUCTIONS

Have the participant perform approximately 15 repetitions of the overhead squat, utilizing positioning and movement instructions given in the chapter. Observe the participant from the anterior (front view), and lateral (side view) for five repetitions each. Record the findings on the chart below.

View	Kinetic Chain Checkpoints	Movement Observation	Yes
Anterior	Feet	Turns out	
	Knees	Moves inward	
Lateral	Lumbo-pelvic-hip complex	Excessive forward lean	
		Low back arches	
	Shoulder complex	Arms fall forward	

Pushing and Pulling

Observe a client/participant either during a session or on the gym floor performing pushing and/or pulling movements.

1. Record your movement observation findings on the following charts.

2. Based on the observed postural compensations, record which muscles might be in a tight position and weak position.

OBSERVATIONAL FINDINGS

Exercise: _____

Kinetic Chain Checkpoints	Movement Observation	Yes
Lumbo-pelvic-hip complex	Low back arches	
Shoulder complex	Shoulders elevates	
Head	Head protrudes while pulling	

Exercise: _____

Kinetic Chain Checkpoints	Movement Observation	Yes
Lumbo-pelvic-hip complex	Low back arches	
Shoulder complex	Shoulders elevates	
Head	Head protrudes while pulling	

CHAPTER 5 — ANSWER KEY

Exercise 5-1 Answers

1. E	3. J	5. C	7. G	9. A
2. H	4. F	6. B	8. D	10. I

6

Flexibility Training Concepts

STUDY GUIDE EXERCISES

Exercise 6-1: Essential Vocabulary

First, skim through Chapter 6 of the text. Then, fully read through Chapter 6 and watch the presentation for Chapter 6. As you read, find and highlight the vocabulary words numbered below.

   The purpose of this exercise is to have an understanding of key terms utilized in the section. Without referring back to the text, match the terms with their proper definitions.

VOCABULARY WORDS

1. _____ Muscle imbalance

2. _____ Altered reciprocal inhibition

3. _____ Autogenic inhibition

4. _____ Golgi tendon organ

5. _____ Muscle spindle

6. _____ Synergistic dominance

7. _____ Flexibility

8. _____ Relative flexibility

DEFINITION

A. Normal soft-tissue extensibility that allows full range of motion of a joint and has optimum control.

B. Where the kinetic chain seeks the path of least resistance during movement.

C. Alterations of lengths of muscles surrounding a joint.

D. When a tight psoas decreases the neural drive to the gluteus maximums, this is an example of?

E. The body's substitution system when there is a weak or inhibited prime mover.

F. Sensory organ of muscle sensitive to length and rate of change of length.

G. Process that stimulates the Golgi Tendon Organ and produces an inhibitory effect on the muscle spindle.

H. Sensory organ sensitive to changes in muscular tension and rate of change of tension.

Exercise 6-2: Short Answer

Review the information in Chapter 6. Now, answer the following questions in one or two sentences.

CORRECTIVE FLEXIBILITY

1. What is the purpose of corrective flexibility?

   _____

   _____

2. What are the two stretching techniques utilized in corrective flexibility?

   _____

   _____

ACTIVE FLEXIBILITY

3. What is the purpose of active flexibility?

   _____

   _____

4. What are the two stretching techniques utilized in active flexibility?

   _____

   _____

FUNCTIONAL FLEXIBILITY

5. What is the purpose of functional flexibility?

   _____

   _____

6. What are the two stretching techniques utilized in functional flexibility?

   _____

   _____

View	Checkpoint	Compensation	Probable Overactive Muscles	Probable Underactive Muscles
Anterior	Feet	Turns Out	Soleus Lat. Gastrocnemius Biceps Femoris (short head)	Med. Gastrocnemius Med. Hamstring Gracilis Sartorius Popliteus
	Knees	Move Inward	Adductor Complex Biceps Femoris (short head) TFL Vastus Lateralis	Gluteus Medius/Maximus Vastus Medialis Oblique (VMO)
Lateral	LPHC	Excessive Forward Lean	Soleus Gastrocnemius Hip Flexor Complex Abdominal Complex	Anterior Tibialis Gluteus Maximus Erector Spinae
		Low Back Arches	Hip Flexor Complex Erector Spinae Latissimus Dorsi	Gluteus Maximus Hamstrings Intrinsic Core Stabilizers (transverse abdominis, multifidus, transversospinalis, internal oblique pelvic floor muscles)
	Upper Body	Arms Fall Forward	Latissimus Dorsi Teres Major Pectoralis Major/Minor	Mid/Lower Trapezius Rhomboids Rotator Cuff
		Shoulders Elevate (Pushing/Pulling Assessment)	Upper Trapezius/Scalenes Levator Scapulae	Mid/Lower Trapezius Rhomboids Rotator Cuff
		Forward Head (Pushing/Pulling Assessment)	Upper Trapezius/Scalenes Levator Scapulae	Deep Cervical Flexors

Exercise 6-3: The OPT Method

INSTRUCTIONS

Column A. List muscles that are in a shortened position, based upon the movement compensation in questions 1 and 2 below (use above table as a reference).

Column B. Pick which stretching technique you would choose for the type of flexibility you are doing.

Column C. List the specific stretch you would do for the short muscles. Utilize stretches given in the chapter.

Column D. Record recommended acute variables for that stretch.

1. The client's feet turn out during an overhead squat assessment. You are designing a Phase 1 program in the stabilization level of the OPT™ Model.

   What type of flexibility training will this require?

   _____

Fill out the following chart, based on the instructions above:

A Short Muscles	B Technique	C Stretch	D Acute Variables

After completion of this chart, practice the stretching techniques (that you wrote with the recommended acute variables) on yourself.

2. The client's arms fall forward during an overhead squat assessment. You are designing a Phase 3 program in the strength level of the OPT™ model.

   What type of flexibility training will this require?

   _____

Fill out the following chart, based on the instructions above:

A Short Muscles	B Technique	C Stretch	D Acute Variables

After completion of this chart, practice the stretching techniques (that you wrote with the recommended acute variables) on yourself.

Exercise 6-4: Observation

For each of the following distortions, find and observe at least one gym member who exhibits these traits. Then, choose which stretching techniques you would employ for that person, if he/she were your client.

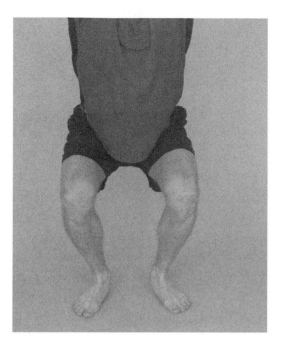

Observations details:

_____

_____

_____

List one stretch you would choose for a client in corrective flexibility who exhibited this deviation:

_____

Technique:

_____

Acute Variables:

_____

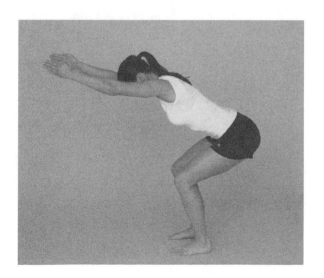

Observations details:

_____

_____

_____

List one stretch you would choose for a client in corrective flexibility, who exhibited this deviation:

_____

Technique:

_____

Acute Variables:

_____

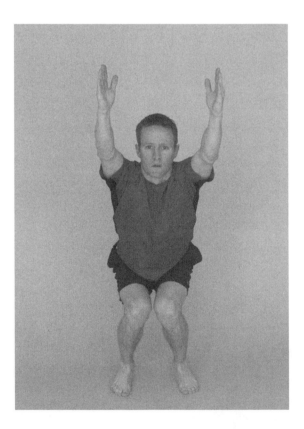

Observations details:

_____

_____

List one stretch you would choose for a client in corrective flexibility, who exhibited this deviation:

_____

Technique:

_____

Acute Variables:

_____

CHAPTER 6 — ANSWER KEY

Exercise 6-1 Answers

1. C	3. G	5. F	7. A
2. D	4. H	6. E	8. B

Exercise 6-2 Answers

1. Corrective flexibility improves muscle imbalances and altered joint motion.
2. **Technique:** Self-myofascial Release
   Description: Roll gently on the muscle until you find a tender area and then hold it for 20–30 seconds.
   Technique: Static Stretching
   Description: Lengthen the muscle to the first point of tension in a noncompensated position and then hold it for 20 seconds.
3. Active flexibility improves extensibility of soft-tissue and increases neuromuscular efficiency through the use of reciprocal inhibition.
4. **Technique:** Self-myofascial Release
   Description: Roll gently on the muscle until you find a tender area and then hold it for 20–30 seconds.
   Technique: Active-isolated Stretching
   Description: Contract the muscle opposite to the one you are stretching and hold it for 2–4 seconds. Repeat 5–10 times.
5. Functional flexibility improves multiplanar extensibility, with optimum neuromuscular control, throughout the entire range of motion.
6. **Technique:** Self-myofascial Release
   Description: Roll gently on the muscle until you find a tender area and then hold it for 20–30 seconds.
   Technique: Dynamic Stretching
   Description: Utilizing your muscles to take you through proper movement.

Exercise 6-3 Answers

1. **Feet turn out:** Corrective Flexibility

A Short Muscles	B Technique	C Stretch	D Acute Variables
Gastrocnemius	Self-myofascial Release Static	Gastrocnemius	1–2 sets, hold 20–30 sec.
Soleus	Self-myofascial Release Static	Soleus	1–2 sets, hold 20–30 sec.
Bicep Femoris (short head)	Self-myofascial Release Static	Bicep femoris	Hold tender areas for 20–30 sec.

2. **Arms fall forward:**

A Short Muscles	B Technique	C Stretch	D Acute Variables
Pectoralis Major	Self-myofascial Release Static Stretching	Pectoral Wall Stretch	1–2 sets, hold 2–4 sec, 5–10 reps
Latissimus Dorsi	Self-myofascial Release Static Stretching	Latissimus Dorsi Ball Stretch	Hold tender areas for 20–30 sec

Exercise 6-4 Answers

1. **Observation:** Feet turn out
   Stretch: Gastrocnemius Stretch
   Technique: Self-myofascial release and static stretching
   Acute Variables: 1–2 sets, hold 20–30 seconds.
2. **Observation:** Excessive Forward Lean
   Stretch: Hip Flexor Complex
   Technique: Self-myofascial release and static stretching
   Acute Variables: 1–2 sets, hold 20–30 seconds.
3. **Observation:** Knees move inward
   Stretch: Standing Adductor Stretch
   Technique: Self-myofascial release and static stretching
   Acute Variables: 1–2 sets, hold 20–30 seconds.

Cardiorespiratory Training Concepts

STUDY GUIDE EXERCISES

Exercise 7-1: Essential Vocabulary

First, skim through Chapter 7 of the text. Then, fully read through Chapter 7 and watch the presentations for Chapter 7. As you read, find and highlight the vocabulary words numbered below.

The purpose of this exercise is to have an understanding of key terms utilized in the section. Without referring back to the text, match the terms with their proper definitions.

VOCABULARY WORDS	DEFINITION
1. _____ Integrated Cardiorespiratory training	A. Consists of movements that more closely mimic those of the actual activity.
2. _____ General warm-up	B. State where the body's metabolism is elevated following exercise.
3. _____ Specific warm-up	C. The number of training sessions for a given time period.
4. _____ Cool-down	D. Point when the body can no longer produce enough energy for the muscles with normal oxygen intake.
5. _____ Frequency	E. Provides body with a smooth transition back to a steady state.
6. _____ Intensity	F. Level of demand the activity places on the body.
7. _____ EPOC	G. Training that involves and places stress on the cardiorespiratory system.
8. _____ Stage training	H. Where intensities are varied throughout the workout.
9. _____ Anaerobic threshold	I. Three-stage programming system that uses different heart training zones.
10. _____ Interval training	J. Preparing the body for physical activity by doing movements that are not specific to the activity to be performed.

Exercise 7-2: True or False

After reading through the chapter, answer True or False to each statement. If the statement is false, write an explanation of why it is false.

1. A warm-up should fatigue the body for an activity before it begins.
   True
   False

   _____

   _____

2. If a first-time client exhibits an anterior pelvic tilt, starting him on a stationary bike or stepper would be best for his cardiorespiratory training.
   True
   False

   _____

   _____

Exercise 7-3: Short Answer

After reading through the chapter, write a brief answer for each of the following questions.

1. What type of flexibility would be most appropriate in the cool-down? Why?

   _____

   _____

2 What is an indictor that a client is ready to move from Stage One to Stage Two in the cardiorespiratory training program?

   _____

   _____

3. Which two stages of training utilizes interval training?

   _____

   _____

4. When designing a program for a client who is in the strength level of the OPT™ model, which two stages should be rotated during the week for the client's cardiorespiratory training?

   _____

   _____

5. When designing a program for a client who is in the power level of the OPT™ model, which stages should be rotated during the week for the client's cardiorespiratory training?

   _____

   _____

Exercise 7-4: OPT™ Method Key Terms

Review the Cardiorespiratory Training Modalities section in Chapter 7. Then complete the following chart. Record the Zone(s) and intensity that the client should be at, which should coincide with the minutes of the workout.

OPT™ Level	Stage	Time	Intensity	Zone	Progression
Stabilization	I	30–60 min.			Time
Strength	II	5–10 min. 1 min. 1 min. Repeat			Increase workload (speed, incline, level, etc.)
Power	III	10 min. 2 min. 1 min. * 1 min. 1 min. 10 min.			Further increase workload

*If the client is unable to drop to the appropriate heart rate during this 1 minute break, stay in Zone Two or Zone One for the rest of the workout.

CHAPTER 7 — ANSWER KEY

Exercise 7-1 Answers

1. G	3. A	5. C	7. B	9. D
2. J	4. E	6. F	8. I	10. H

Exercise 7-2 Answers

1. False. A warm-up should prepare the body for activity. Fatiguing can lead to altered muscle recruitment and detract from the purpose of proper training.
2. False. Bikes and/or steppers may not be best, as the hips are placed in a constant state of flexion, adding to a shortened hip flexor complex.

Exercise 7-3 Answers

1. Corrective. This type of flexibility accomplishes the goals of a cool-down, which are to relax the muscles and bring them back to their original length.
2. The client can maintain a Zone One heart rate for at least 30 minutes two to three times per week.
3. Stage II and III
4. Stage I, Stage II
5. Stage I, Stage II, Stage III

Exercise 7-4 Answers

OPT™ Level	Stage	Time	Intensity	Zone	Progression
Stabilization	I	30–60 min.	65%–75%	One	Time
Strength	II	5-10 min. 1 min. 1 min. Repeat	65%–75% 80%–85% 65%–75%	One Two One	Increase workload (speed, incline, level, etc.)
Power	III	10 min. 2 min. 1 min. * 1 min. 1 min. 10 min.	65%–75% 80%–85% 86%–90% 80%–85% 86%–90% 65%–75%	One Two Three Two Three One	Further increase workload

Core Training Concepts

STUDY GUIDE EXERCISES

Exercise 8-1: Essential Vocabulary

First, skim through Chapter 8 of the text. Then, fully read through Chapter 8 and watch the presentations for Chapter 8. As you read, find and highlight the vocabulary words numbered below.

The purpose of this exercise is to have an understanding of key terms utilized in the section. Without referring back to the text, match the terms with their proper definitions.

VOCABULARY WORDS

1. _____ Core

2. _____ Intramuscular coordination

3. _____ Intermuscular coordination

4. _____ Drawing-in maneuver

DEFINITION

A. Ability of the neuromuscular system to allow muscles to work together with proper activation and timing between them.

B. Pulling the region just below the navel toward the spine.

C. Ability of the neuromuscular system to allow optimal levels of motor unit recruitment and synchronization within a muscle.

D. The lumbo-pelvic-hip complex, thoracic, and cervical spine.

Exercise 8-2: True or False

After reading Chapter 8, answer True or False to each statement. If the statement is false, write an explanation of why it is false.

1. The musculature of the core is divided into two categories: the stabilization system and the movement system.
   True
   False

2. The movement system is responsible for the stability of the lumbo-pelvic-hip complex.
   True
   False

3. The stabilization system is responsible for the movement of the core.
   True
   False

4. When working optimally, each structural component of the core distributes weight, absorbs force, and transfers ground-reaction forces.
   True
   False

5. A weak core can lead to predictable patterns of injury.
   True
   False

After reviewing the Implementing a Core Training Program section of Chapter 8, fill in the empty blocks in the table below. Check your answers before progressing to the next exercise.

Exercise 8-3: OPT™ Method Key Terms

Core Systems	OPT™ Level	Phase(s)	Exercise	Number of Exercises	Sets	Reps	Tempo	Rest
Stabilization	Stabilization	1	Core Stabilization	1–4	1–3		Slow (4/2/1)	0–90 sec.
Movement	Strength	2 3 4	Core Strength	0–4	2–3	8–12		0–60 sec.
Movement	Power	5	Core Power			8–12	As fast as can be controlled	0–60 sec.

Exercise 8-4: Practical Application

LESSON ONE

Review the exercise descriptions in Chapter 8 and practice each stabilization level exercise. Perform 10–25 repetitions using a slow (4/2/1) tempo. Most importantly, be sure to use perfect form.

STABILIZATION LEVEL EXERCISES

1. Marching

2. Floor Prone Cobra

3. Prone Iso-ab

4. Floor Bridge

LESSON TWO

Next, practice each strength level exercise. Perform 8–12 repetitions using a 3-2-1 tempo. Most importantly, be sure to use perfect form.

STRENGTH LEVEL EXERCISES

1. Ball Crunch

2. Reverse Crunch

3. Back Extension

4. Cable Rotation

LESSON THREE

Last, practice each power level exercise. Perform 10 repetitions, using a fast yet controlled tempo. Most importantly, be sure to use perfect form.

POWER LEVEL EXERCISES

1. Rotation Chest Pass

2. Ball Medicine Ball Pullover

3. Front Med Ball Oblique Throw

4. Woodchop Throw

CHAPTER 8 — ANSWER KEY

Exercise 8-1 Answers

1. D   3. A
2. C   4. B

Exercise 8-2 Answers

1. True
2. False. The movement system is responsible for movement of the core.
3. False. The stabilization system is responsible for stabilization of the core.
4. True
5. True

Exercise 8-3 Answers

Core Systems	OPT™ Level	Phase(s)	Exercise	Number of Exercises	Sets	Reps	Tempo	Rest
Stabilization	Stabilization	1	Core Stabilization	1–4	1–3	**12–20**	Slow (4/2/1)	0–90 sec.
Movement	Strength	2 3 4	Core Strength	0–4	2–3	8–12	**Medium (3/2/1–1/1/1)**	0–60 sec.
Movement	Power	5	Core Power	**0–2**	**2–3**	8–12	As fast as can be controlled	0–60 sec.

Balance Training Concepts

STUDY GUIDE EXERCISES

Exercise 9-1: Essential Vocabulary

First, skim through Chapter 9 of the text. Then, fully read through Chapter 9 and watch the presentations for Chapter 9. As you read, find and highlight the vocabulary words numbered below.

The purpose of this exercise is to have an understanding of key terms utilized in the section. Without referring back to the text, match the terms with their proper definitions.

VOCABULARY WORDS

1. _____ Dynamic joint stabilization

2. _____ Multisensory condition

3. _____ Controlled instability

4. _____ Limit of stability

DEFINITION

A. Training environment that provides heightened stimulation to proprioceptors and mechanoreceptors.

B. The distance outside of an individual's base of support that he/she can go without losing control of their center of gravity.

C. Training environment that is as unstable as can safely be controlled by an individual.

D. Ability of the kinetic chain to stabilize a joint during movement.

Exercise 9-2: True or False

After reading through Chapter 9, answer True or False to each statement. If the statement is false, write an explanation of why it is false.

1. Balance is a static process.
   True
   False

2. Adequate force reduction and stabilization are required for optimum force production.
   True
   False

_____

3. An individual's limit of stability is the distance outside of the base of support that he/she can go to, without losing control of his/her center of gravity.
   True
   False

_____

4. Only when playing sports is balance training effective.
   True
   False

_____

5. Maintenance of postural equilibrium is a static process.
   True
   False

_____

6. The main goal of balance training is to continually increase the client's awareness of his/her limits of stability by creating the most unstable environment available.
   True
   False

_____

Exercise 9-3: Practical Application

LESSON ONE

Review the exercise descriptions in Chapter 9 and practice each stabilization level exercise. Perform 10 repetitions on each leg while holding each repetition 3 seconds in perfect alignment.

STABILIZATION LEVEL EXERCISES

1. Single-leg Balance

2. Single-leg Balance Reach

3. Single-leg Balance Hip Internal and External Rotation

4. Single-leg Lift and Chop

LESSON TWO

Next, practice each strength level exercise. Perform 8 repetitions on each leg while moving through a tempo of 3-2-1 in perfect alignment.

STRENGTH LEVEL EXERCISES

1. Single-leg Squat

2. Single-leg Squat Touchdown

3. Single-leg Romanian Deadlift

4. Step-up to Balance

5. Lunge to Balance

LESSON THREE

Last, practice each power level exercise. Perform 8 repetitions on each leg while moving through a controlled tempo and holding the "land" position for 3 seconds.

POWER LEVEL EXERCISES

1. Multiplanar Hop with Stabilization
   a. Sagittal Plane Hop with Stabilization
   b. Frontal Plane Hop with Stabilization
   c. Transverse Plane Hop with Stabilization

2. Box Hop-up with Stabilization

3. Box Hop-down with Stabilization

Exercise 9-4: OPT™ Method Key Terms

After reviewing Chapter 9, fill in the empty blocks in the table below. Check your answers before progressing to the next exercise.

OPT™ Level	Phase(s)	Exercise	Number of Exercises	Sets	Reps	Tempo	Rest
Stabilization	1	Balance-stabilization exercises		1–3	12–20 (or single-leg, 6–10 each)	Slow (4/2/1)	0–90 sec.
Strength	2 3 4	Balance-strength exercises	0–4	2–3	8–12		0–60 sec.
Power	5	Balance-power exercises	0–2	2–3		Controlled (Hold the landing position for 3–5 seconds).	

CHAPTER 9 — ANSWER KEY

Exercise 9-1 Answers

1. D 3. C

2. A 4. B

Exercise 9-2 Answers

1. False. Functional balance is a dynamic process involving multiple neurological pathways.
2. True
3. True
4. False. Whether on a basketball court, stability ball, or walking down stairs, maintaining balance is the key to all functional movements.
5. False. Postural equilibrium is an integrated, dynamic process requiring optimal muscular balance, joint dynamics, and neuromuscular efficiency.
6. False. The main goal of balance training is to increase a client's limits of stability by training in the most unstable environment that he/she can safely control.

Exercise 9-4 Answers

OPT™ Level	Phase(s)	Exercise	Number of Exercises	Sets	Reps	Tempo	Rest
Stabilization	1	Balance-stabilization exercises	**1–4**	1–3	12–20 (or single-leg, 6–10 each)	Slow (4/2/1)	0–90 sec.
Strength	2 3 4	Balance-strength exercises	0–4*	2–3	8–12	**Medium (3/2/1–1/1/1)**	0–60 sec.
Power	5	Balance-power exercises	0–2**	2–3	**8–12**	Controlled (Hold the landing position for 3–5 seconds).	**0–60 sec.**

Reactive (Power) Training Concepts

STUDY GUIDE EXERCISES

Exercise 10–1: Essential Vocabulary

First, skim through Chapter 10 of the text. Then, fully read through Chapter 10 and watch the presentations for Chapter 10. As you read, find and highlight the vocabulary words numbered below.

The purpose of this exercise is to have an understanding of key terms utilized in the section. Without referring back to the text, match the terms with their proper definitions.

VOCABULARY WORDS	DEFINITION
1. _____ Integrated performance paradigm	A. Exercises that utilize quick, powerful movements involving an eccentric contraction immediately followed by an explosive concentric contraction.
2. _____ Reactive training	B. To move with precision, forces must be reduced (eccentrically), stabilized (isometrically) and then produced (concentrically).
3. _____ Rate of force production	C. Ability of the muscles to exert maximal force output in a minimal amount of time.

Exercise 10–2: Practical Application

LESSON ONE

Review the exercise descriptions in Chapter 10 and practice each stabilization level exercise. Perform 8 repetitions, while holding each repetition 3 seconds, in perfect alignment.

STABILIZATION LEVEL EXERCISES

1. Squat Jump with Stabilization

2. Box Jump-up with Stabilization

3. Box Jump-down with Stabilization

4. Horizontal Jump with Stabilization

LESSON TWO

Next, practice each strength level exercise. Perform 5–10 repetitions while repeating each repetition as fast as can be controlled.

STRENGTH LEVEL EXERCISES

1. Squat Jump

2. Tuck Jump

3. Butt Kick

4. Power Step-up

LESSON THREE

Last, practice each power level exercise. Perform 5 repetitions, while repeating each repetition as fast as can be controlled.

POWER LEVEL EXERCISES

1. Ice Skater

2. Single-leg Power Step-up

3. Proprioceptive Plyometrics

Exercise 10-3: OPT™ Method Key Terms

After reviewing Chapter 10, fill in the empty blocks in the table below. Check your answers before progressing to the next exercise.

OPT™ Level	Phase(s)	Exercise	Number of Exercises	Sets	Reps	Tempo	Rest
Stabilization	1	Reactive-stabilization exercises	0–2	1–3		Controlled (Hold stabilization position for 3–5 seconds)	0–90 sec.
Strength	2 3 4	Reactive-strength exercises		2–3	8–10		0–60 sec.
Power	5	Reactive-power exercises	0–2		8–12	As fast as possible	0–60 sec.

CHAPTER 10 — ANSWER KEY

Exercise 10-1 Answers

1. B   2. A   3. C

Exercise 10-3 Answers

OPT™ Level	Phase(s)	Exercise	Number of Exercises	Sets	Reps	Tempo	Rest
Stabilization	1	Reactive-stabilization exercises	0–2	1–3	**5–8**	Controlled (Hold stabilization position for 3–5 seconds)	0–90 sec.
Strength	2 3 4	Reactive-strength exercises	**0–4**	2–3	8–10	**Medium (Repeating)**	0–60 sec.
Power	5	Reactive-power exercises	0–2	**2–3**	8–12	As fast as possible	0–60 sec.

Speed, Agility, and Quickness Training Concepts

STUDY GUIDE EXERCISES

Exercise 11-1: Essential Vocabulary

First, skim through Chapter 11 of the text. Then, fully read through Chapter 11 and watch the video presentations for Chapter 11. As you read, find and highlight the vocabulary words numbered below.

The purpose of this exercise is to have an understanding of key terms utilized in the section. Without referring back to the text, match the terms with their proper definitions.

VOCABULARY WORDS

1. _____ Speed

2. _____ Agility

3. _____ Quickness

DEFINITION

A. The ability to react to stimulus and change the motion of the body in all planes of motion.

B. The ability to accelerate, decelerate, and change direction quickly, while maintaining proper posture.

C. The ability to move the body in one intended direction as fast as possible.

Exercise 11-2: Short Answer

Review the information in Chapter 11. Now, answer the following questions in one or two sentences.

1. Speed is the product of _____ and _____.

   Define each answer in your own words.

a: _____

b: _____

2. Proper sprint mechanics includes frontside mechanics (which involves _____) and backside mechanics (which involves _____).

   Describe each answer in your own words.

   a: _____

   b: _____

Exercise 11-3: OPT™ Method Key Terms

OPT™ Level	Phase(s)	SAQ Exercise	Sets	Reps	Rest
Stabilization	1	___ speed ladder drills	1–2	Half ladder	0–60 sec.
		___ cone drills	1–2		0–90 sec.
Strength	2	___ speed ladder drills	3–4	Half ladder	0–60 sec.
	3				
	4	1–2 cone drills	2–3		0–90 sec.
Power	5	6–9 speed ladder drills	3–6	Half ladder	0–60 sec.
		___ cone drills	3–6		0–90 sec.

Exercise 11-4: Practical Application

Review the exercise descriptions in Chapter 11 and practice each SAQ Speed Ladder Drill and Cone Drill exercise, utilizing the guidelines from Exercise 11-3.

Remember: All exercises should be performed with precise techniques and kinetic chain control to minimize risk of injury. Exercise execution should also be taken into account, if applicable in current environment.

LESSON ONE: SAQ SPEED LADDER DRILLS

1. One-ins

2. Two-ins

3. Side shuffle

4. In-in/Out-out

5. Side In-in/Out-out

6. In-in-out (Zigzag)

7. Ali Shuffle

LESSON TWO: SAQ CONE DRILLS

1. 5-10-5 Drill

2. Box Drill

3. T-Drill

4. L.E.F.T. Drill

CHAPTER 11 — ANSWER KEY

Exercise 11-1 Answers

1. C   2. B   3. A

Exercise 11-2 Answers

1. Speed is the product of stride rate and stride length.
   a. Stride rate is the number of strides taken in a given amount of time.
   b. Stride length is the distance covered in one stride.
2. Proper sprint mechanics includes frontside mechanics (which involves triple flexion) and backside mechanics (which involves triple extension).
   a. Triple flexion includes ankle dorsiflexion, knee flexion, and hip flexion of the front leg.
   b. Triple extension includes the actions of ankle plantar flexion, knee extension, and hip extension of the back leg.

Exercise 11-3 Answers

OPT™ Level	Phase(s)	SAQ Exercise	Sets	Reps	Rest
Stabilization	1	**4–6** speed ladder drills **1–2** cone drills	1–2 1–2	Half ladder	0–60 sec. 0–90 sec.
Strength	2 3 4	**6–9** speed ladder drills 1–2 cone drills	3–4 2–3	Half ladder	0–60 sec. 0–90 sec.
Power	5	**6–9** speed ladder drills **2–4** cone drills	3–6 3–6	Half ladder	0–60 sec. 0–90 sec.

Resistance Training Concepts

STUDY GUIDE EXERCISES

Exercise 12-1: Essential Vocabulary

First, skim through Chapter 12 of the text. Then, fully read through Chapter 12 and watch the presentations for Chapter 12. As you read, find and highlight the vocabulary words numbered below.

The purpose of this exercise is to have an understanding of key terms utilized in the section. Without referring back to the text, match the terms on the left with their proper definitions, on the right.

VOCABULARY WORDS

1. _____ General Adaptation Syndrome

2. _____ Alarm Reaction

3. _____ Resistance Development

4. _____ Exhaustion

5. _____ Periodization

6. _____ Principle of Specificity

7. _____ Mechanical Specificity

8. _____ Neuromuscular Specificity

9. _____ Metabolic Specificity

10. _____ Strength

DEFINITION

A. Stress that is intolerable to the client and that will produce breakdown or injury.

B. Principle that states the body will specifically adapt to the type of demand placed upon it.

C. Refers to the energy demand placed upon the body.

D. The ability of the neuromuscular system to produce internal tension to overcome external force.

E. General pattern of adaptation brought forth by stresses placed upon the kinetic chain.

F. The initial reaction to a stressor that allows for protective processes within the body.

G. A stage where the kinetic chain increases its functional capacity to adapt to the stressor.

H. Refers to the speed of contraction and exercise selection.

I. Refers to the weight and movements placed on the body.

J. Division of a training program into smaller, progressive stages.

Exercise 12-2: Adaptations

STABILIZATION LEVEL

1. What are the two primary adaptations achieved in this period of training?

   _____

2. Describe the first adaptation in one sentence.

   _____

3. Describe the second adaptation in one sentence.

   _____

4. Circle one of the following choices in each row below that best describes the variables used to achieve the adaptations in the stabilization level.

   Repetitions: High Low

   Volume: Low/Moderate Moderate/High

   Intensity: Low/Moderate Moderate/High

   Exercises: Stable Controlled Unstable High Velocity

STRENGTH LEVEL EXERCISES

5. What are the three primary adaptations achieved in this period of training?

   _____

6. Describe the first adaptation in one sentence.

   _____

7. Describe the second adaptation in one sentence.

   _____

8. Describe the third adaptation in one sentence.

   _____

9. Circle one of the following choices in each row below that best describes the variables used to achieve the adaptations in the strength level.

   Repetitions: Low/Moderate High

   Volume: Low/Moderate Moderate/High

   Intensity: Low/Moderate Moderate/High

   Exercises: Stable Controlled Unstable High Velocity

POWER LEVEL EXERCISES

10. What is one primary adaptation achieved in this period of training?

_____

11. Describe that adaptation in one sentence.

_____

12. Circle one of the following choices in each row below that best describes the variables used to achieve the adaptations in the power level.

Intensity: Low/Moderate Moderate/High Low/High

Exercises: Stable Controlled Unstable High Velocity

CHAPTER 12 — ANSWER KEY

Exercise 12-1 Answers

1. E	3. G	5. J	7. I	9. C
2. F	4. A	6. B	8. H	10. D

Exercise 12-2 Answers

STABILIZATION LEVEL

1. Muscular endurance and stability.
2. The ability to maintain relatively low levels of force over prolonged periods of time.
3. The ability of the kinetic chain's stabilizing muscles to provide optimal dynamic joint stabilization and maintain correct posture during all movements.
4. Repetitions: High

   Volume: Low/Moderate

   Intensity: Low/Moderate

   Exercises: Controlled Unstable

STRENGTH LEVEL

5. Strength endurance, hypertrophy, and maximal strength.
6. The ability to repeatedly produce high levels of force for prolonged periods of time.
7. Enlargement of muscle fibers in response to increased volumes of tension.
8. The maximum force that a muscle can produce in a single, voluntary effort, regardless of how fast the load moves.
9. Repetitions: Low/Moderate

   Volume: Moderate/High

   Intensity: Moderate/High

   Exercises: Stable

POWER LEVEL

10. Power.
11. The ability to produce the greatest possible force in the shortest possible time.
12. Intensity: Low/High

    Exercises: High Velocity

Program Design

STUDY GUIDE EXERCISES

Exercise 13-1: Essential Vocabulary

First, skim through Chapter 13 of the text. Then, fully read through Chapter 13 and watch the presentations for Chapter 13. As you read, find and highlight the vocabulary words below.

   The purpose of this exercise is to have an understanding of key terms utilized in the section.

1. Without referring back to the text, write the appropriate definition for each term in your own words.

   Repetition:

   _____

   _____

   Set:

   _____

   _____

   Repetition Tempo:

   _____

   _____

   Training Intensity:

   _____

   _____

   Rest Interval:

   _____

   _____

Training Volume:

_____

_____

Training Frequency:

_____

_____

Training Duration:

_____

_____

2. Fill in the blanks with the correct word from the list below. Hint: Words can be used more than once.

Greater

After

3–5

Fewer

Before

Energy supplies

Slow

Higher

Rest periods

Explosive

Lower

Proprioception

Moderate

60–90

Tempo

a. The heavier the load the _____ the number of repetitions.

b. The individual usually performs _____ sets when performing higher repetitions at a lower intensity and _____ sets when performing lower repetitions at a higher intensity.

c. For the goal of stabilization, a _____ repetition tempo will be utilized. For the goal of power, an _____ repetition tempo will be utilized. For strength adaptations, a _____ repetition tempo will be utilized.

d. Training intensity should be determined _____ sets and repetitions. Other ways to alter intensity besides just external resistance are _____, _____, and _____.

e. By adjusting the rest interval _____ can be regained according to the goal of the program.

f. High intensity programs should be at _____ volumes to help ensure a safe training program.

g. Optimum training frequency for improvements in strength is _____ times per week.

h. Programs that exceed_____ minutes are associated with rapidly declining energy levels.

Exercise 13-2: OPT™ Method Key Terms

Review the information in Chapter 13. Now, fill in the blanks in the following chart.

Period of Training (Main Adaptation)	Specific Adaptation	Phases Used	Phase Name	Exercise Type (Stabilization, Strength or Power)	Method of Progression
Stabilization	Endurance Stability	1 2		Stabilization	
Strength	Strength Endurance Hypertrophy Maximal Strength				Volume Load
Power	Power	6 7			Speed

Exercise 13-3: OPT™ Method Application

In this exercise, a client scenario is given and the assessment process is provided. Following the instructions listed below, design the most appropriate individualized program for this client.

INSTRUCTIONS

1. Read the client profile, including the subjective and objective information. The assessment information (physiological and movement) is provided.

2. Design an annual, monthly, and weekly plan based upon the client information.

3. Complete a fitness program for the first workout with this client. Hint: Use the preceding study guide chapters to assist with each component of the program.

   Brief Client Summary

   Name: Mrs. Rossini

   Goals: Be healthy, decrease body fat, and be pain free.

   Dedication: Mrs. Rossini is able to dedicate 3 days per week to her training program.

Training History: Mrs. Rossini has never been on a training program before.

Age: 51

Height: 5'4"

Weight: 135

Body Fat %: 30%

Blood Pressure: 120/80

Resting Heart Rate: 80

Step Test Result: 40

Client's Occupation

	Questions	Yes	No
1	What is your current occupation? *School Teacher*		
2	Does your occupation require extended periods of sitting?		N
3	Does your occupation require extended periods of repetitive movements? (If yes, please explain.) *Half of the day is spent sitting and the other half is spent moving around with the children*	Y	
4	Does your occupation require you to wear shoes with a heel (dress shoes)?		N
5	Does your occupation cause you anxiety (mental stress)?	Y	

Lifestyle

	Questions	Yes	No
1	Do you partake in any recreational activities (golf, tennis, skiing, etc.)? (If yes, please explain.) _____ _____		
2	Do you have any hobbies (reading, gardening, working on cars, etc.)? (If yes, please explain.) _____ _____		

Physical Activity Readiness Questionnaire (PAR-Q)

	Questions	Yes	No
1	Has your doctor ever said that you have a heart condition and that you should only perform physical activity recommended by a doctor?		N
2	Do you feel pain in your chest when you perform physical activity?		N
3	In the past month, have you had chest pain when you were not performing any physical activity?		N
4	Do you lose your balance because of dizziness or do you ever lose consciousness?		N
5	Do you have a bone or joint problem that could be made worse by a change in your physical activity?		N
6	Is your doctor currently prescribing any medication for your blood pressure or for a heart condition?		N
7	Do you know of any other reason why you should not engage in physical activity?		N

Medical History

	Questions	Yes	No
1	Have you ever had any pain or injuries (ankle, knee, hip, back, shoulder, etc.)? (If yes, please explain.) **_Experiences knee pain_**	Y	
2	Have you ever had any surgeries? (If yes, please explain.)		N
3	Has a medical doctor ever diagnosed you with a chronic disease, such as coronary heart disease, coronary artery disease, hypertension (high blood pressure), high cholesterol, or diabetes? (If yes, please explain.)		N
4	Are you currently taking any medication? (If yes, please list.)		N

Overhead Squat Assessment

View	Kinetic Chain Checkpoints	Movement Observation	Yes
Anterior	Feet	Turn out	Y
	Knees	Move inward	Y
Lateral	Lumbo-pelvic-hip complex	Excessive forward lean	
		Low back arches	Y
	Shoulder complex	Arms fall forward	

Annual Plan

	Phase	JAN	FEB	MAR	APR	MAY	JUN	JUL	AUG	SEP	OCT	NOV	DEC
Stab.	1												
Strength	2												
	3												
	4												
Power	5												
Cardio													

Monthly Plan

Week	1							2							3							4						
Day	M	T	W	T	F	S	S	M	T	W	T	F	S	S	M	T	W	T	F	S	S	M	T	W	T	F	S	S
Phase 1																												
Phase 2																												
Phase 3																												
Phase 4																												
Phase 5																												
Cardio																												

CHAPTER 13 — ANSWER KEY

Exercise 13-1 Answers

1. **Repetition:** One complete movement of a particular exercise.
   Set: A group of consecutive repetitions.
   Repetition Tempo: Speed with which each repetition is performed.
   Training Intensity: An individual's level of effort compared to his/her maximum effort.
   Rest Interval: Time taken between sets and/or exercises.
   Training Volume: Total amount of work performed within a specified time period.
   Training Frequency: The number of training sessions that are performed during a specified period (usually 1 week).
   Training Duration: Timeframe from the start of the workout to the finish, including the warm-up and cool-down or the length of time spent in one phase of training.

2.
   a. Fewer
   b. Fewer, greater
   c. Slow, explosive, moderate
   d. After, proprioception, rest periods, tempo
   e. Energy supplies
   f. Lower
   g. 3–5
   h. 60–90

Exercise 13-2 Answers

Annual Plan

	Phase	JAN	FEB	MAR	APR	MAY	JUN	JUL	AUG	SEP	OCT	NOV	DEC
Stab.	1	x		x		x		x		x		x	
Strength	2		x		x		x		x		x		x
	3												
	4												
Power	5												
Cardio		x	x	x	x	x	x	x	x	x	x	x	x

Monthly Plan

Week					1							2							3							4			
Day	M	T	W	T	F	S	S	M	T	W	T	F	S	S	M	T	W	T	F	S	S	M	T	W	T	F	S	S
Phase 1	x		x		x			x		x		x			x		x		x			x		x		x		
Phase 2																												
Phase 3																												
Phase 4																												
Phase 5																												
Cardio	x		x		x			x		x		x			x		x		x			x		x		x		

Exercise 13-3 Answers

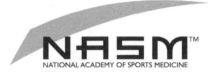

OPT For Fitness

Name: Mrs. Rossini	Month: 1
Date: 08/10/06	Week: 1
Professional: Scott Lucett	Day: 1 of 12

Program Goal:
PHASE 1: FAT LOSS

STEP 1

A. Foam Roll

Foam Roll	Sets	Duration
Calves	1	30 sec.
IT Band	1	30 sec.
Adductors	1	30 sec.

B. Stretch

Static Stretching	Sets	Duration
Wall Calf Stretch	1	30 sec.
Standing Psoas Stretch	1	30 sec.
Standing Adductor Stretch	1	30 sec.

C. Cardiovascular

Treadmill	5-10 min.

STEP 2

A. Core

Exercise	Sets	Reps	Tempo	Rest
Floor Bridge	2	15	Slow	0
Floor Prone Cobra	2	15	Slow	0

B. Balance

Exercise	Sets	Reps	Tempo	Rest
Single-leg Balance	2	X	Slow	60

C. Reactive

Exercise	Sets	Reps	Tempo	Rest
Optional – until she has better core strength and balance				

STEP 3

Resistance Training Program

Body Part	Exercise	Sets	Reps	Intensity	Tempo	Rest
Total Body	Ball Squat, Curl to Press	2	15	60%	Slow	0
Chest	Ball Dumbbell, Chest Press	2	15	60%	Slow	0
Back	Standing Cable Row	2	15	60%	Slow	0
Shoulder	Standing Dumbbell Scaption	2	15	60%	Slow	0
Biceps	Optional					
Triceps	Optional					
Legs	Front Step Up to Balance	2	15	60%	Slow	90 sec

STEP 4

Cool Down

Repeat Steps 1A and/or 1B

Special Populations

STUDY GUIDE EXERCISES

Exercise 14-1: Essential Vocabulary

First, skim through Chapter 14 of the text. Then, fully read through Chapter 14 and watch the presentations for Chapter 14. As you read, find and highlight the vocabulary words numbered below.

The purpose of this exercise is to have an understanding of key terms utilized in the section. Without referring back to the text, match the terms with their proper definitions.

VOCABULARY WORDS

1. _____ Obesity

2. _____ Diabetes

3. _____ Hypertension

4. _____ Osteopenia

5. _____ Osteoporosis

6. _____ Arthritis

7. _____ Osteoarthritis

8. _____ Rheumatoid arthritis

9. _____ Cancer

10. _____ Restrictive lung disease

11. _____ Obstructive lung disease

DEFINITION

A. Condition in which there is a decrease in bone mass and density as well as an increase in the space between bones.

B. Degenerative joint disease in which the body's immune system mistakenly attacks its own tissues.

C. Condition where lung tissue is normal, but flows are restricted.

D. Characterized by narrowing of the major arteries that are responsible for supplying blood to the lower extremity.

E. Degeneration of cartilage in joints.

F. Fastest growing health problem in the United States.

G. The precursor to osteoporosis and is indicated by lowered bone mass.

H. Condition where the ability to expand the lungs is decreased.

I. Metabolic disorder in which the body's ability to produce insulin or to utilize glucose is altered.

J. Characterized by limping, lameness, and/or pain in the lower leg during mild exercise, resulting from a decrease in blood to the lower extremities.

K. Blood pressure of 140/90 or greater.

12. _____ Intermittent claudication

13. _____ Peripheral arterial disease

L. Any various types of malignant neoplasm, most of which invade surrounding tissues, may spread to several sites, and are likely to recur after attempted removal.

M. Inflammatory condition that mainly affects the joints.

Exercise 14-2: Self Check

After reading through Chapter 14, check your understanding of key concepts by answering the following questions.

List three physiological differences between children and adults. Explain each difference in one or two sentences.

1. _____

_____

2. _____

_____

3. _____

_____

Exercise 14-3: Self Check

After reading through Chapter 14, check your understanding of key concepts by answering the following questions.

List three considerations to take into account when designing a program for an obese client. Briefly explain how this may affect exercise selection.

1. _____

2. _____

3. _____

List the two types of diabetes. Briefly describe each type in one or two sentences.

4. _____

5. _____

List one recommendation that may need to be avoided when working with Type II diabetic clients. Explain why in one sentence.

6. _____

Exercise 14-4: Self Check

Fill in the blanks with the correct word from the list below. Hint: Words can be utilized more than once.

Femur	Peripheral	Twelve
Third	Heart action	Bone mass
One	Supine	Moderate
Two	Estrogen	Lumbar
Three	Prone	Peak bone mass
Body position	Circuit	

1. When training the hypertensive client, it is imperative that the fitness professional also monitor _____. _____ or _____ positions can increase tension.

2. Phase _____ would be appropriate for a population experiencing hypertension. Programs can be performed in a _____ style and/or using the ____ ____ ____ training system.

3. A principal observation in Type I osteoporosis is a deficit in _____.

4. Osteoporosis mainly affects the neck of the _____ and _____, which are structures considered part of the core.

5. One of the most important risk factors that influences osteoporosis is _____. This is the highest amount of _____ a person is able to achieve during his/her lifetime.

6. Guidelines for individuals with osteoporosis include Phases _____ and _____ of the OPT™ model.

7. With regard to pregnant clientele, those engaged in an exercise program prior to pregnancy may continue with _____ levels of exercise until the _____ trimester.

8. As the pregnant client progresses to more advanced stages of pregnancy or after _____ week(s), performing exercises in a prone or supine position is not advised.

Exercise 14-5: Self Check

List five contraindications for self-myofascial release as it relates to special populations. Hint: Examples include type of special population and/or clients who have specific conditions.

1. _____

2. _____

3. _____

4. _____

5. _____

CHAPTER 14 — ANSWER KEY

Exercise 14-1 Answers

1. F	5. A	8. B	11. C
2. I	6. M	9. L	12. J
3. K	7. E	10. H	13. D
4. G			

Exercise 14-2 Answers

1. Peak oxygen uptake. The term "maximum oxygen uptake" should not be utilized to describe peak assessed values in children, because children do not exhibit a plateau in oxygen uptake at maximum exercise.
2. A lower absolute sweating rate contributes to children having less of a tolerance to temperature extremes.
3. Lower glycolytic enzymes seen in children decrease their ability to perform high intensity or anaerobic tasks for prolonged periods of time.

Exercise 14-3 Answers

1. Due to lack of balance and stepping parameters balance or proprioceptive training may better facilitate the obese individual rather than strength training alone.
2. Utilize exercises from a standing or seated position. There is a high probability that obese clients will exhibit hypertension or high blood pressure. Be cautious when placing a client in a prone or supine position.
3. Engage in weight supported exercises to decrease orthopedic stress.
4. Type I—Impairs normal glucose management. Blood sugar is not optimally delivered to the cells resulting in hyperglycemia (high levels of blood sugar). To control this, Type I diabetics must inject insulin to compensate for what they cannot produce.
5. Type II—There is an ability to produce adequate amounts of insulin, but cells are resistant to the insulin. The cells do not allow insulin to bring adequate amounts of blood sugar into the cell.
6. Weight bearing activity needs to be avoided to prevent blisters and micro-trauma that could result in foot infection.

Exercise 14-4 Answers

1. Body position, supine, prone
2. Phase 1, circuit, Peripheral Heart Action
3. Estrogen
4. Femur, vertebrae
5. Peak bone mass, bone mass
6. Phases 1 and 2
7. Moderate, third trimester
8. 12 weeks

Exercise 14-5 Answers

1. It is contraindicated for the hypertensive population, because it requires lying down.
2. It is contraindicated for the client who has osteoporosis.
3. For the pregnant client, avoid self-myofascial on the inside of the lower leg, as this may be linked to premature uterine contraction.
4. It is contraindicated for the client who has varicose veins.
5. It is contraindicated for the client who has intermittent claudication, unless approved by licensed physician.

Nutrition

STUDY GUIDE EXERCISES

Exercise 15-1: Essential Vocabulary

First, skim through Chapter 15 of the text. Then, fully read through Chapter 15 and watch the presentations for Chapter 15. As you read, find and highlight the vocabulary words numbered below.

The purpose of this exercise is to have an understanding of key terms utilized in the section. Without referring back to the text, match the terms with their proper definitions.

VOCABULARY WORDS

1. _____ Nutrition

2. _____ Protein

3. _____ Essential amino acids

4. _____ Nonessential amino acids

5. _____ Biological value

6. _____ Protein synthesis

7. _____ Complete protein

8. _____ Incomplete protein

9. _____ Gluconeogenesis

DEFINITION

A. Amino acids the body is able to manufacture.

B. The utilization of protein for building and repairing tissues or structures.

C. The sum of processes by which an animal or plant takes in and utilizes food substances.

D. A food source that is low or lacking in one or more essential amino acids.

E. Amino acids are utilized to assist in energy production.

F. Made up of amino acids linked together by peptide bonds.

G. Amino acids the body is unable to manufacture.

H. A measure of protein quality or how well it satisfies the body's essential amino acids needs.

I. A food source that supplies all of the essential amino acids in appropriate ratios.

Exercise 15-2: Processes

Place the following events of protein digestion and absorption in their proper sequence.

a. Protein fragments leave the stomach and enter into the small intestine where they continue to be dismantled.

b. Singular amino acids are absorbed through the intestinal wall and released into the blood supply to the liver.

c. Ingested proteins enter the stomach.

d. Pepsin cleaves the protein strand into smaller stands of several amino acids.

e. Hydrochloric acid uncoils the protein leading to the dismantling peptide bonds.

1. _____

_____

2. _____

_____

3. _____

_____

4. _____

_____

5. _____

_____

Exercise 15-3: Self Check

List three negative side effects associated with high protein diets.

1. Side Effect: _____

2. Side Effect: _____

3. Side Effect: _____

Exercise 15-4: Self Check

Fill in the blanks with the correct word from the list below. Hint: Words can be used more than once.

Fats	Energy intake
10%–30%	Carbohydrates
Oils	Fat
96	50%–70%
60%	Glycemic index
Unsaturated	Saturated
Glycogen	

a. The storage form of carbohydrates in humans is _____.

b. The rate at which ingested carbohydrates raise blood sugar and its accompanying effect on insulin release is referred to as _____.

c. Weight gain or loss is related to total _____, not the source of food eaten.

d. The limiting factor for exercise performance is _____ availability because maximal _____ utilization cannot occur without it.

e. For most moderately active adults, a carbohydrate intake between _____ is recommended.

f. For individuals participating in endurance exercise a diet consisting of _____ of total calories from carbohydrates is recommended.

g. Of the lipids contained in foods, 95% are _____ and _____.

h. _____ fatty acids are implicated as a risk factor for heart disease by raising bad cholesterol levels, whereas _____ fats are associated with increases in good cholesterol.

i. If the goal is fat loss or to enhance overall health, a diet containing _____ of calories from fat is recommended.

j. An individual should drink approximately _____ ounces of water per day.

Exercise 15-5: Self Check

List two attributing factors that a low carbohydrate diet has on weight loss.

1. Attributing factor: _____

2. Attributing factor: _____

CHAPTER 15 — ANSWER KEY

Exercise 15-1 Answers

1. C	3. G	5. H	7. I	9. E
2. F	4. A	6. B	8. D	

Exercise 15-2 Answers

1. c
2. e
3. d
4. a
5. b

Exercise 15-3 Answers

1. Side Effect: Calcium depletion
2. Side Effect: Fluid imbalance
3. Side Effect: It can contribute to risk factors for heart disease and some types of cancer.

Exercise 15-4 Answers

a. Glycogen
b. Glycemic index
c. Energy intake
d. Carbohydrates, fat
e. 50%–70%
f. 60%
g. Fats, oils
h. Saturated, unsaturated
i. 10%–30%
j. 96

Exercise 15-5 Answers

1. Attributing factor: Low caloric intake
2. Attributing factor: Loss of fat-free mass

16

Supplementation

STUDY GUIDE EXERCISES

Exercise 16-1: Essential Vocabulary

First, skim through Chapter 16 of the text. Then, fully read through Chapter 16 and watch the presentations for Chapter 16. As you read, find and highlight the vocabulary words numbered below.

The purpose of this exercise is to have an understanding of key terms utilized in the section. Without referring back to the text, match the terms with their proper definitions.

VOCABULARY WORDS

1. _____ Dietary supplement

2. _____ Dietary Reference Intakes

3. _____ Estimated Average Requirement

4. _____ Recommended Dietary Allowance

5. _____ Adequate Intake

6. _____ Tolerable Upper Intake Level

7. _____ Supplement facts panel

DEFINITION

A. Provides guidelines for what constitutes an adequate intake of a nutrient.

B. A recommended average daily nutrient intake level based on estimates of nutrient intake that are adequate for group(s) of healthy people.

C. Labels that provide product information on required nutrient amounts and percent of daily value.

D. The average daily intake level that is sufficient to meet the nutrient requirement of nearly all healthy individuals.

E. A substance that completes or makes an addition to daily intake.

F. The average daily nutrient intake level that is estimated to meet the requirement of half the healthy individuals who are in a particular life stage and gender group.

G. The highest average daily nutrient intake level likely to pose no adverse health effects to almost all individuals.

Exercise 16-2: Processes

Complete the following sentences with the appropriate vitamin and/or mineral from the given list.

Vitamin K   Iron

Vitamin D   Magnesium

Folic acid   Vitamin A

Vitamin E

1. Upper Intake Level values are set for each nutrient except for _____ and _____. The ULs for these nutrients are set from supplements or pharmacological sources only.

2. Excess _____ can cause birth defects when a woman is taking too much at conception and during early pregnancy.

3. Excess _____ can result in the calcification of blood vessels and eventually damage the function of kidneys, heart, and lungs.

4. Excess intake of _____ can interfere with the absorption of other minerals and can cause gastrointestinal irritation.

5. Supplementation with vitamin E and _____ can complicate conditions for people on blood thinners.

6. Large doses of anti-inflammatory drugs may interfere with _____ function and increase its requirement.

CHAPTER 16 — ANSWER KEY

Exercise 16-1 Answers

1. E	3. F	5. B	7. C
2. A	4. D	6. G	

Exercise 16-2 Answers

1. Vitamin E, magnesium
2. Vitamin A
3. Vitamin D
4. Iron
5. Vitamin K 150
6. Folic acid

Behavior Modification

STUDY GUIDE EXERCISES

Exercise 17-1: Essential Vocabulary

First, skim through Chapter 17 of the text. Then, fully read through Chapter 17 and watch the presentations for Chapter 17. Without referring back to the text, match the steps with their definitions.

STEPS

1. _____ Step One   _____ Vision

2. _____ Step Two   _____ Strategy

3. _____ Step Three   _____ Belief

4. _____ Step Four   _____ Persistence

5. _____ Step Five   _____ Learning

DEFINITIONS

A. The process of working hard toward goal(s) and rebounding from setbacks.

B. One of the most powerful predictors of change and success.

C. Being certain about what one wants from life.

D. Involves self-monitoring, which simply means recording aspects of behavior and measuring progress toward goals.

E. Properly setting personal goals through the process of strategy refinement.

Exercise 17-2: Short Answer

Review Chapter 17 and then answer the following questions in your own words.

1. List three benefits to asking "why" questions.

   a. _____

   b. _____

   c. _____

2. List three reasons why properly setting goals is important.

   a. _____

   b. _____

   c. _____

3. If a health and fitness professional had a client that was expressing negative thoughts during a training session, what would be one thing the fitness professional could do to help the client battle the negativity?

   _____

   _____

4. List three ways that a health and fitness professional can help his/her client to persist in an exercise program. Describe each in one or two sentences.

   a. _____

   _____

   b. _____

   _____

   c. _____

   _____

CHAPTER 17 — ANSWER KEY

Exercise 17-1 Answers

1. C   3. B   5. D
2. E   4. A

Exercise 17-2 Answers

1. a. "Why" questions allow the health and fitness professional to be better equipped to customize fitness programs.
   b. They more effectively motivate clients by reminding them of their ultimate ambitions.
   c. They communicate the benefits of additional sessions more persuasively.

2. a. Setting goals properly channels effort.
   b. Setting goals boosts motivation.
   c. Setting goals enhances performance.
3. The health and fitness professional can "schedule" negativity by setting aside time for self-doubt. Remind the client that there will be plenty of time to plague himself or herself at that scheduled time, but not during the session.
4. a. Reward success by giving clients a self-reward system that makes instant gratification a positive force for change.
   b. Facilitate networks of excellence. Encourage clients to ask for support from friends and family.
   c. Have a strategy for setbacks. Prepare clients to expect success, but prepare for setbacks by using strategies such as calling a friend or having a "reminder card."

Professional Development

STUDY GUIDE EXERCISES

Exercise 18-1: Essential Concepts

First, skim through Chapter 18 of the text. Then, fully read through Chapter 18 and watch the presentations for Chapter 18. Without referring back to the text, answer the following questions in one or two sentences, using your own words.

1. What does uncompromising customer service mean to you?

_____

_____

2. List three ways that you, personally, can provide uncompromising customer service.

   a. _____

   b. _____

   c. _____

Exercise 18-2: Essential Concepts

Fill in the appropriate answers to the following question.

1. List five ways that a health and fitness professional can approach potential clients.

   a. _____

   b. _____

c. _____

d. _____

e. _____

Exercise 18-3: Essential Concepts

Answer the following questions:

1. What does the acronym READ stand for?

   R _____

   E _____

   A _____

   D _____

In your own words, define each step in the READ system in one or two sentences.

2. R _____

   E _____

   A _____

   D _____

3. Building rapport with a potential client involves three factors. What are they?

   a. _____

   b. _____

   c. _____

Exercise 18-4: Understanding Features and Benefits

Read each of the following scenarios. Then, answer the question that follows it in one or two sentences as if speaking to a client. Hint: Refer to Table 18-1 for help.

1. Client Scenario: Mr. Jones wants to lose weight and tone.
   Question: What are the benefits of Mr. Jones performing the flexibility, core, balance, and reactive components of his program?
   Answer:_____

2. Client Scenario: Mrs. Rossini wants to increase hypertrophy and gain strength.
   Question: What are the benefits of Mrs. Rossini performing stabilization level resistance training exercises?
   Answer:_____

Exercise 18-5: Application for Success Questions.
You may need to use a calculator.

Utilizing the 10-step process, complete the following

1. What is your annual income goal?

   _____

2. What is your weekly income goal?

   _____

3. How many sessions need to be performed per week?

   _____

4. What is your closing percentage?

   _____

5. In what timeframe do you want to acquire new clients?

   _____

6. How many potential clients need to be contacted overall?

   _____

7. How many potential clients need to be contacted each day?

   _____

8. How many potential clients need to be contacted hourly?

   _____

9. Will you ask each member for their contact information?

   _____

10. How do you follow up?

   _____

Start recording your steps to success. In the given time period you have chosen, complete the given chart with contacts and follow-up information as you progress onward in your career as a health and fitness professional.

Contact Name	Date of First Contact	Card Sent	First Call	Second Call	Assessment Date	Show?	Result	Follow-up Action Plan

CHAPTER 18 — ANSWER KEY

Exercise 18-1 Answers

1. Uncompromising customer service means being adamant about providing an experience and level of assistance that is rarely, if ever, experienced anywhere else.
2. a. Take every opportunity to meet and greet each club member at all times.
   b. Never give the impression that any question is inconvenient.
   c. Do not merely receive complaints, but take ownership of them.

Exercise 18-2 Answers

1. a. Say "Hello!" to every member while working on shift.
   b. Offer very active members a towel or water if the club has it available.
   c. Simply introduce yourself by name and ask members for their names as well.
   d. Let members know that you are there to enrich the club experience by attending to their needs. Then do it!
   e. Let your first interaction with a member be nonthreatening by resisting the temptation to educate. Be pleasant and professional.

Exercise 18-3 Answers

1. Rapport, Empathy, Assessment, Developing
2. Rapport is essential in the beginning phases of the relationship between the fitness professional and the client. It is characterized by similarity, agreement, or congruity. Empathy is understanding and identifying with the thoughts and feelings of another. Assessment is the process of determining the importance or value of something allowing for direct focus into the client and his/her specific needs. Developing involves designing a program and having the ability to demonstrate how each component of the OPT™ model relates to the client's wants, goals, and needs.
3. a. Establish trust.
    b. Have effective communication.
    c. Create a confident, enthusiastic, and professional presence.

Exercise 18-4 Answers

1. The benefit to performing flexibility, core, balance, and reactive training in her program will allow for greater tone in target areas. Also, a potential for greater activation of desired muscles and increased caloric expenditure.
2. The benefit to performing stabilization level resistance training exercises is it will allow greater joint stabilization, which will permit greater activation of muscles and force production.